Longevity Training-Book 9-Avoiding Accidents

This book is a transcription and reproduction of the training course materials from Course #9 "Avoiding Accidents"

When all of your other long term health issues are covered, then the biggest danger of dying becomes Accidents.

Since I've had so many premonition experiences I've learned a lot about how they work and am confident we can all learn how to see the probability of the future ourselves.

The information and exercises in this book should help you to avoid dangerous situations in your future and therefore be safer and live longer.

Our spirit exists outside of time and space and by observing from the core spirit we can do amazing things!

Longevity Training-Book 9-Avoiding Accidents

Longevity Training-Book 9-Avoiding Accidents

Copyright Page

The book is copyrighted for 2018

Longevity Training-Book 9-Avoiding Accidents

By Martin K. Ettington

Longevity Training-Book 9-Avoiding Accidents

Other books by Martin K. Ettington

Longevity Training-Book 9-Avoiding Accidents

Strange and Ancient Places in the USA
A Theory of Ancient Prehistory And
    Giant Aliens
<u>Aliens and Space</u>
Aliens and Secret Technology
Aliens Are Already Among Us
Designing and Building Space Colonies
Humanity and the Universe

All About Moon Bases
All About Mars Journeys and Settlement
The Space and Aliens Six Books Bundle
A Theory of Ancient Prehistory and
    Giant Aliens
The Space Colonies and Space
    Structures Coloring Book
All About Asteroids

<u>The Longevity Training Series</u>

(A transcription of the online Multimedia Longevity Coaching Training Program)

The Personal Longevity Training Series-Book1-Long Lived Persons
The Personal Longevity Training Series-Book2-Your Soul's Purpose
The Personal Longevity Training Series-Book3-Enable Your Life Urge
The Personal Longevity Training Series-Book4-Your Spiritual Connection
The Personal Longevity Training Series-Book5-Having Love in Your Heart
The Personal Longevity Training Series-Book6-Energy Body Health
The Personal Longevity Training Series-Book7-The Science of Longevity
The Personal Longevity Training Series-Book8-Physical Body Health
The Personal Longevity Training Series-Book9-Avoiding Accidents
The Personal Longevity Training Series-Book10-Implementing These Principles

The Personal Longevity Training Series-Books One Thru Ten

These books are all available in digital and printed formats from my
website and on Amazon, Barnes & Noble, Apple ITunes, and many other sites

My Books Website is: http://mkettingtonbooks.com

Longevity Training-Book 9-Avoiding Accidents

<u>Signup for our Mailing List to get the following:</u>

1) A discount coupon for 25% discount on all books on our site

2) Occasional Notices of new books available

3) Occasional Email on other offerings of ours (Monthly)

Go to this link to sign-up:

http://personal-longevity.com/mkebooks/emailsignup/

And click this link to get the FREE 102 page Ebook titled "Secrets of Many Things"

If you have any questions about this book or other subjects please contact the Author at:

mke@mkettingtonbooks.com

Longevity Training-Book 9-Avoiding Accidents

Table of Contents

Introduction

Back in 2008 I became very interested in the field of Longevity and Physical Immortality. After a lot of research this led me to my first book on the subject "Physical Immortality: A History and How to Guide". This book was pretty popular and I wanted to continue learning about Longevity and what things we could do about it in our lives.

The subject continued to fascinate me to the point that I developed a Longevity Coaching program over a couple of years starting in 2011. This online training program was multimedia—consisting of videos, my writings on longevity to read, online exercises, and tests for each of ten courses. It also included a lot of additional resources for each course including extra courses on how to become a successful Longevity Coach. A student who completed the training and tests successfully would become certified as a "Longevity Coach" and authorized to teach this material to others.

I developed a set of ten principles on longevity which are as follows:

The 10 Principles of Personal Longevity are:

- The Reality of Long Lived People
- Defining Your Purpose in Life
- Enabling the Life Urge
- Your Spiritual Health
- Having Love in Your Heart
- Energy Body Health
- The Science of Longevity
- Physical Body Health
- Using your Intuition for Safety
- Implementation of these principles

What are the 10 Principles all about?

The Reality of Long Lived People

The first principle is where I provide lots of evidence of people who have lived well over the age of 120 years old to 150-180-200, and even a 256 year old man from China:

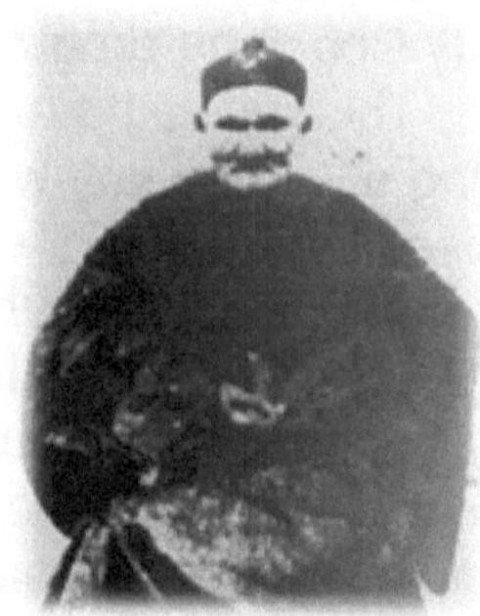

LI CHING-YUN: The Longest Lived person of record-256 Years (Source-The New York Times-May 6, 1933)

The Second Principle of Life Purpose

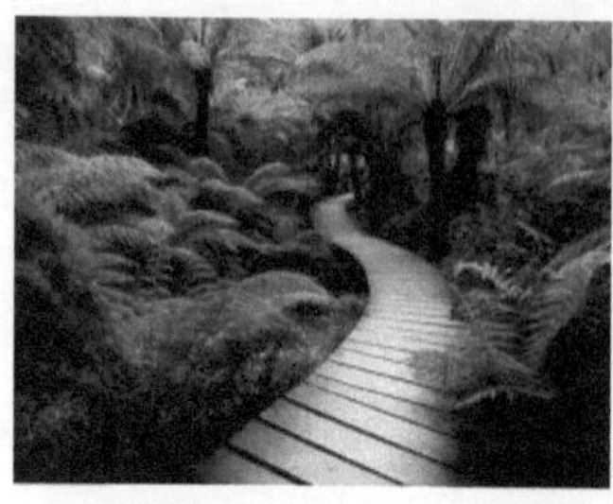

One of the things that occurred to me when I was putting the 10 principles together was that if one doesn't have a reason to live, or purpose in life--then what is the point?

This meant I had to add a very important step of how you can develop your own life purpose, or bring it up to date with your phase in life. Without reviewing your purpose-- then none of the rest of the principles matter.

Enabling the Life Urge

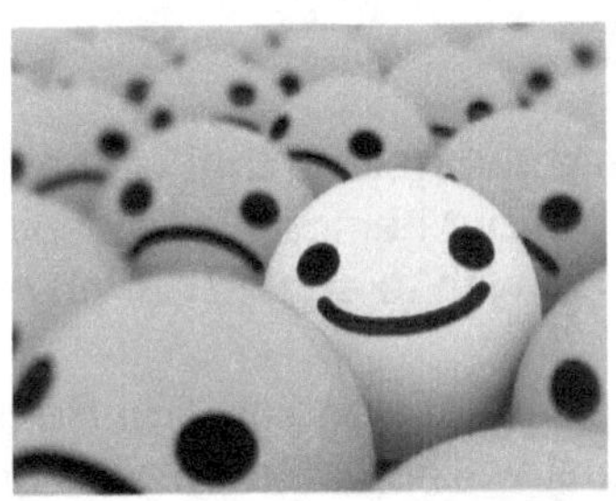

Have you ever realized how we are all programmed to expect to live through certain stages in life and then die? It's so common in our society that we don't think it odd that we expect to die at a certain age?

Have you ever heard radio ads saying "You are getting up in your sixties and seventies" so it's time to come out to our cemetery and buy a plot"

How ridiculous is this? And do you see how much our subconscious has been programmed towards death?

This principle is all about reprogramming ourselves to have a more positive outlook on life and its possibilities.

Having a Spiritual Connection in Your Life

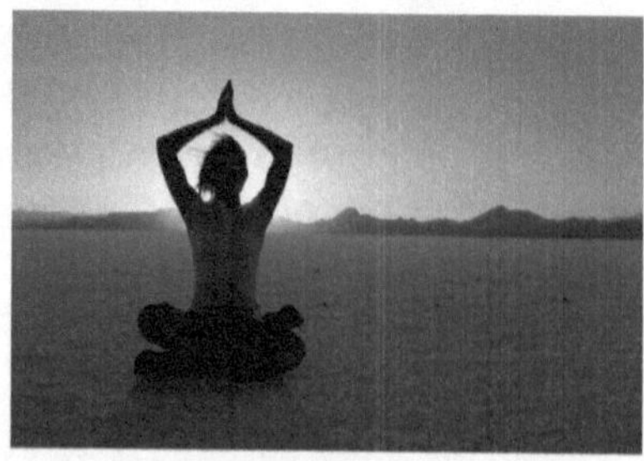

Most of us innately understand that we have a spiritual core in the center of our being. It is this spiritual core that we need to connect with to enable our physical health too.

It doesn't matter what religion you are. Regular meditation, deep prayer, or just walking in the woods helps you make and keep that connection in your life.

Having Love in Your Heart

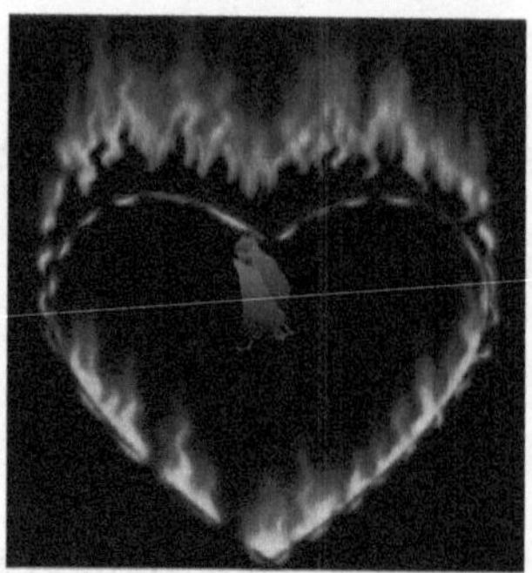

One of the most important things I learned in the last five years was that Unconditional Love is a real and physical thing. It is a powerful energy force in life and not just a philosophical belief system.

I considered it so important that I added it as a separate principle of longevity.

True Unconditional Love is healing, embodies happiness, and is a powerful part of our vital forces.

Energy Body Health

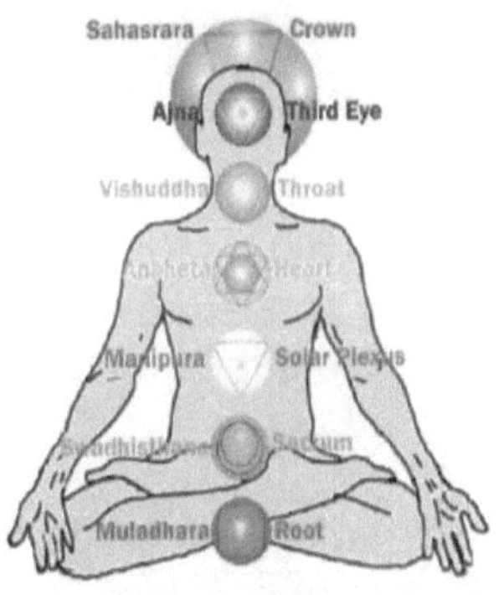

We all have an energy body which is part of our vital forces. The Indians talk about the "Chakras" and the Chinese talk about "Energy Meridians" in Acupuncture.

We should all learn different practices to keep our vital forces flowing for maximum health and vitality.

The Science of Longevity

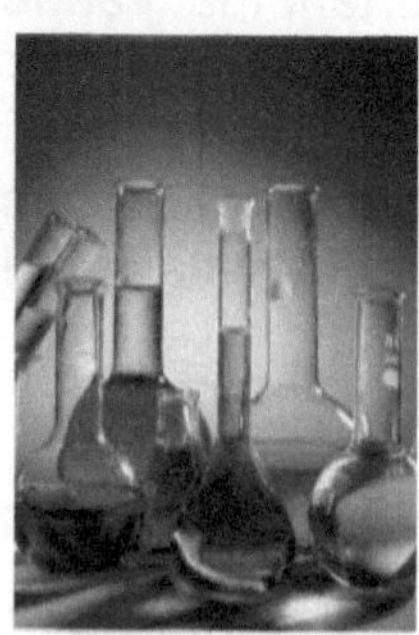

Science and Medicine are making new discoveries all the time that we can take advantage of to extend our lives. Why not take advantage of these discoveries which provide new therapies and supplements to increase our longevity.

There is also a lot we can learn from plants and animals. We all share the same genetic basis.

Some of these plants and animals live thousands of years and some cells are immortal.

What can we learn from them to apply to our lives?

Physical Body Health

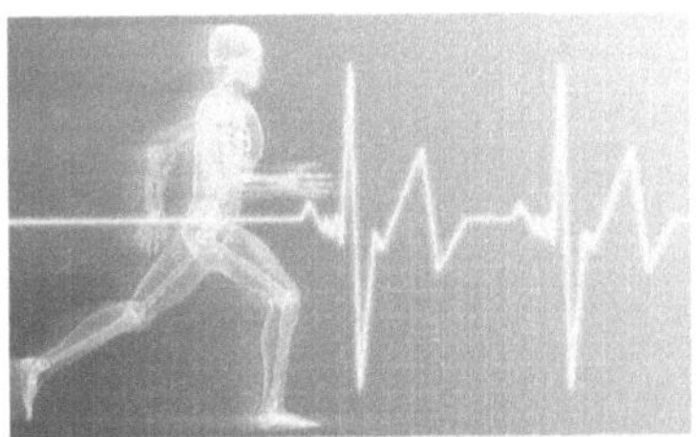

There are many types of supplements used for anti-aging for thousands of years. What can we learn about them that we can apply to our lives?

What other considerations about our physical health does nontraditional or alternative medicine offer?

Using Your Intuition for Safety

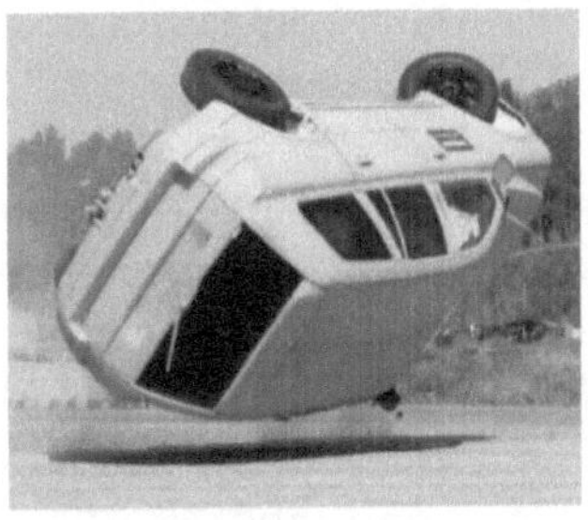

Once you have established your own long term health then what is the greatest danger you face?

ACCIDENTS

We can learn to use our intuition to make us safer as well as see potential future events which may be good too.

Why not open up to the possibilities of how our spirit has this natural ability in all of us?

Implementing These Principles in Your Life

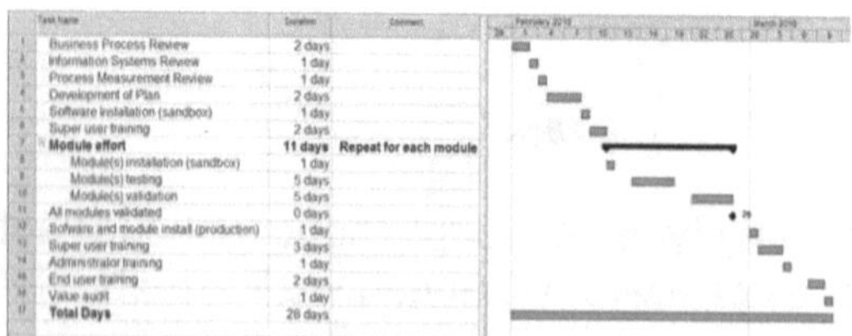

It's nice to read about all these concepts, but how can you really apply them to your own life?

This is what the chapter on implementation is all about, and it helps you plan a lifelong change in your health focus to live these principles and truly experience long term health, greater happiness, and extended longevity.

For five years I amended and improved these materials which now include a lot more information and helpful concepts for students wanting to improve their longevity and those of others.

I transcribed my videos and other materials to this book so you can read it all, and later hear it in an AudioBook.

This book is priced pretty inexpensively, compared to the online training and certification program which sells in total for $1,995 USD. If you are interested in taking the entire online program at a major discount, then please contact me at:

Marty@personal-longevity.com

Hope you enjoy these materials since when applied correctly they will significantly change your life.

PLP Concepts Overview

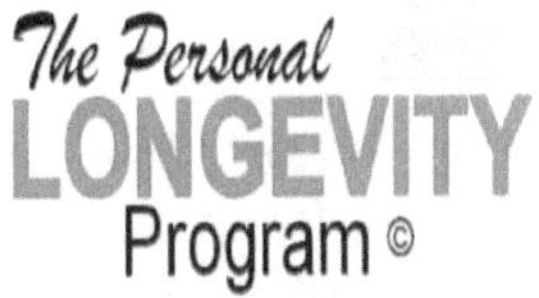

(Transcription of overview video)

Hello I'm Martin Ettington and I'd like to introduce you to the Personal Longevity Program which is an integrated holistic approach to long-term health. In this video we will only cover the high level concepts which comprise individual courses in the coaching certificate program for personal longevity.

The first concept is that long lived people exist and have existed for hundreds of thousands of years. We cover in the first course all about their records; along with people not only in places you might think like India, but in Europe and the United States-people who've lived long lives and well documented cases.

We discuss people who have lived well over the age of 120 and even the case of a Chinaman who lived to 256 years old. Plus a lot of mythology about people who have lived even longer lives so you get an idea that extending your life much longer than we think is currently medically and scientifically possible is certainly something that can happen.

The second course's concept has to do with finding your souls purpose. The point of wanting to live a long life is to know what your purpose in life is, so we go through some readings and some exercises to help you determine where soul's purpose in life is. Then doing goals as a fundamental concept so you will know the motivations in your life.

Third is the "Psychology of Living" also known by certain practitioners as "Removing the death Urge". The psychology of living has to do with seeking a positive image about your ability to live a long time. We tend to be programmed from birth about the idea that we are going to go through certain stages in our life as a child, as a teenager, and as adults. It's about reprogramming your subconscious as to the possibilities of a long life.

I've also learned in my life that it is very important to be able open your heart to unconditional love. When you're able to love unconditionally it also helps increase the strength of your immune system and fight off disease. So this is an aspect of spiritual growth. The courses also cover unconditional love and energy body forces. Managing your energy body is an important component of who you are in having energy working properly in your body and is another aspect of health for the length of longevity.

There are many types of scientific and medical research which are being done today and which will contribute to human longevity in the future.

Do you know that the average lifespan in the United States in 1900 was only about 40 years? We have doubled lifespan in the last century with current technologies but things under way in terms of scientific and medical improvements will help extend your lives further.

Also in this course on longevity we will cover a lot of the concepts which are being researched by scientists today. There are suggestions for more things you can do to do to use this science to improve your health along with physical supplements.

A unique thing that I thought about and decided to offer in these courses has to do with all my experiences in prophecy and how I was able to change outcomes on accidents that would occur to me by using simple exercises you can learn to change these outcomes. If you're in great health often the biggest thing you have to worry about are accidents.

We also provide guidelines you can follow on a daily basis and plans you can make to live healthier and happier and have a much longer life than you ever thought possible.

Thank you for listening !

Course #9 Intro Video

(Transcription of Video)

Hello I'm Marty Ettington and this is the introductory video for course number nine of the personal longevity program. This course is titled "Avoiding Accidents" you might ask what does longevity have to do with prophecy? And not a lot specifically but once you're healthy both physically, energy wise, and spiritually, and your body is doing very well then the biggest danger you have towards continued life is accidents.

And as we all know many thousands of accidents kill people all over the country every year, so there's a way to divine your future. And the probability of any accidents happening to you. Why not take advantage of it now? One of the things that I've been very blessed with in my life is I've had a lot of experiences about prophecy both personally and for world events.

And some of these some of these prophecies of mine saved my life. It helped me learn a lot about the probability of the future and it led to an exercise that you're going to learn in this course also about how to avoid accidents. So I'll start with some stories about personal events that had happened to me that helped me learn about how prophecy works. The first one was when I was 19 and I was working at a summer job in an engineering department in upstate New York.

They let me meditate at my desk so I was doing that one day and I was thinking about a trip that I was going to take the Cape Cod for the last couple of weeks after the job was over before school started again and as I was doing that I had a brilliant vision of being on a surfboard that I fell off

when I went under the water came up and the surfboard
came towards me BAM-and hit me in the chin. It knocked
me out of the meditation-I was extremely shocked because
it was so vivid and had just knocked me out of that and I
wondered what it was anyway. A couple weeks later sure
enough I'm walking down the beach in Cape Cod, I
forgotten all about this and I saw some guys with
surfboards so I asked them where I can rent one they said
why don't you come trying with us? So I did it and I spent
all day trying to get up on the board. I wasn't very good at
it. I kept falling off and I got very tired and about two
o'clock in the afternoon I tried to get up again-fell off went
underwater and the same exact scene happens and I
came up and the board hitting the broadside in my chin. I
was all bloody and it almost knocked me out. I had to go to
the hospital and get ten stitches and two sutures in my chin
and I think you cracked my jaw. So it was a pretty nasty
accident and it was the first time in my life that I had this
type of prophecy about something happening to me.

I wondered is it something I could have changed or was it
totally foreordained? Well, I had a lot of other prophecies
over the years but the most significant one is the one that
helped me understand that there is a probability to our
future and then it can be changed through force of will.
This happened in 1998 when I was waiting for a new
contract with Boeing and my family and I were planning on
taking a trip to Spain. My ex-wife's family lived in
Barcelona, but because i thought the contract was
imminent I decided to stay home for a few weeks and see
if I the contract would close.

After a week I found out the contract wasn't going to close
for probably another month so I figured I'd just go ahead
and go to Spain by myself. I decided to try and call the
travel agent to get a reservation as I tried to do that I got a

very dark black feeling and I just couldn't do it. I should also mention at the time that I'd been feeling for a year or two that my life was going to end soon. So anyway I tried the first time I couldn't do it-the second time I tried I got a dark black feeling again. I thought this is really weird and I knew from previous experience that I was getting a warning. The third time I tried actually picked up the phone and again a black feeling of death and so I put it down, It was very strong and I just knew based on my previous experiences that if I went ahead with this flight I would die. But I really wanted to be there because I wanted to be with my family and my young infant son so I had a lot of momentum of a probable route to go to Spain but I knew that that would kill me. So I made a very hard decision which a lot of people would think is nuts and after thinking about it for hours and meditating on I finally decided not to go. I called my wife and told her that I meditated about it and it seemed to me that the day I was going to leave which was September second 1998 that something very bad would happen. So as soon as I made the decision and called her I was very upset about not going but it was like a weight lifted from my mind. Time went by and I was feeling pretty bad and pretty stupid about not going. On September second a Swiss Air flight-that there was a good chance I would have been on-crashed off Newfoundland and everybody on board was killed-several hundred people. So I can't be sure that this would have happened to me but based on my previous experience I know that that was my fate.

Also I should tell you that the premonitions I had about having a short life went away after that point so I really believe that by force of will and making the decision to not go I really changed my future and gave myself many more years in this world.

One more example I'll give you which was not a fatal one but one of the things I often learn to do after that was every time I was going to take a trip somewhere I kind of ran over the trip in my mind to see if there would be good events or bad events-to what would happen. I was doing it for a family trip that we were planning from California to Disney World when I started getting in my mind images of a black dotted line all the way around the Epcot Center. It was kind of dark but it wasn't anything fatal so I decided to go ahead with the trip. To make a long story short I took a ride in Epcot Center-I think it was a trip to Mars-where I got sick to death and had to go to the infirmary for several hours because of motion sickness I had threw up all over everything in the I ride. So now I understand that I was getting a warning that it wouldn't be fatal but then I would have a really nasty time there.

So all of these experiences plus many more I had led me to understand that the probability of the future really exists there are different probable avenues in your future. You can choose which ones you want to take. Some are much more for likely than others but in most cases by force of will you can change what's going to happen to you.

So in this course we are also you're going to be learning more about prophecy, the history of prophecy, different types of prophecy, and fortune-telling from my book: "Prophecy: A history and How to Guide". You're going to learn the avoiding accidents exercise and then there's going to be some more Ebooks you'll read, and some more documents to learn different fortune-telling techniques. Because the more you practice those types of things the better your ability becomes to be able to see the future. The way I see it is our Eternal Spirit is part of the no time, no space, continuum and when we connect with our spirit that allows us to see things outside of time.

Premonitions allows us to see things in the future and that's how prophecy works-by connecting with your eternal spirit. You're able to see probable futures that may happen to you and that's how it works. Thank you very much!

Prophecy: A History and How to Guide

Following are various chapter extracts from my book on Prophecy where I discussed all about my experiences, my theories about how it works, and how you can utilize prophecy yourself.

Chapter 8: Some Personal Stories of Seeing the Future

In this chapter I'm sharing some of my personal experiences.

These experiences provide a basis for my subjective analysis of how prophecy works.

These examples are also intended to show the reader that I do know what I'm talking about when it comes to having "sensed" the future.

a.   Visions

During the summer of 1975 I had a summer CO-OP job at General Electric's Gas Turbine engineering group in Schenectady, NY

At this time I used to meditate at my desk during the lunch hour.

One day in early August I was meditating and thinking about a trip I was planning to Cape Cod. My mind was wandering as I was thinking about what I would do there. My thoughts went to what I would do at the beach.

All of a sudden, I had a blinding flash of a scene where I was in the surf at the beach, and a surfboard was coming towards me. Then a shock occurred and I was thrown out of my meditation and was wide-awake.

I thought that this was pretty weird, and mentioned this to a friend or two.

Two weeks later I was walking on the beach on Cape Cod. I saw a couple of guys with surfboards and asked where I could rent one to give it a try.

They said they had an extra one and I could try it with them.
(I had totally forgotten my vision at this point)

I tried to get up on that board all day, and had some modest success, but I was also getting exhausted in the process.

I decided to try it again and fell off when a big wave hit me. Next thing I knew I was coming up to the surface and I saw the exact same scene from my meditation.

The board hit me hard in the chin and almost knocked me out. I staggered to the shore and the two guys I was with helped me to the hospital where they put 10 stitches and 2 sutures into my chin.

The question arises—Would I have been able to avoid the accident if I had remembered my vision and not gone surfing?

Later experiences have convinced me that the future is a set of probabilities, and we have free will to decide our actions.

I also had an experience on that trip of being able to partially heal my wounds very quickly through a deep meditation and application of psychic healing techniques. However, I do still have a small scar on my chin from this accident.

b.   Warnings of Danger

• Detroit

In 1980 I was moving from Dekalb, Illinois to Rochester, NY between assignments at General Electric, Inc.

While staying with my cousin outside Detroit, I made arrangements one evening to meet an old RPI friend Steve. We decided to go into downtown Detroit to the newly completed Renaissance Center to eat dinner and look around.

The Renaissance Center was built near the water and surrounded by slums.

After dinner we were walking out through the lower level in an area that was all boarded up with nobody else there.

Suddenly, I had this strong urge to turn around and go to find a restroom. I stopped walking forward because the urge was so strong.

I tried to walk forward again and again a very strong urge came to turn around and go back into the main center where other people were.

I remarked to Steve that I couldn't go forward—that something wouldn't let me.

Just then two black guys in trench coats appeared about 30 feet away from behind one of the foundation pillars we were about to walk past.

They started walking towards us with smiles pasted on their faces.

My friend Steve took off running back into the main area and after a moment or two I figured I didn't know what these guys were carrying under their coats, so I ran too.

In less than 30 seconds we were back in a populated area with Police present, and the two guys chasing us gave us smiles like "next time w'ell get you" and took off going the other way.

I had previously always tried to pray to God for protection, and tried to give a subconscious message to my senses to warn me of danger.

I'm convinced that whatever sense or "angel" warned me that evening, I would have been killed or severely wounded if I had continued walking out of the complex with no warning.

Longevity Training-Book 9-Avoiding Accidents

- At the Border in El Paso

In December of 1987 my Dad drove out to Houston to accompany me on my move to Los Angeles where we were going to start a business together.

The first night on the road we stayed overnight in El Paso, Texas near the border.

Sunday morning I suggested we stretch our legs by taking a walk down to the Border which appeared to be less than a mile.

As we were walking through a rundown area near the border I had a strong sense that we were in danger. This sense continued for several minutes that somebody wanted to hurt us.

I told my Dad we needed to turn around and he agreed.

We got back to the hotel safely, and even though we didn't see any danger, I'm convinced my extra senses picked up something.

- Planning a Trip to Spain

During early August of 1998, my wife and I decided to send her and our kids to visit her mother in Barcelona, Spain.

I was going to buy a ticket separately, and meet them there during early September.

When I started to call the travel agent to book my ticket I had a terrible feeling of fear about taking the flight.

I tried two other times to book the ticket during the week for a September 2nd departure, and each time I got the same strong feelings of fear and death.

I have always prayed and tried to guard myself mentally to avoid disasters, so finally I took the warning seriously and decided not to go at all.

This was very difficult to do since I really wanted to see my wife and kids, and this meant I would be home alone for a month.

Work wasn't an excuse either, since I wasn't doing any really heavy contract work at the time and could easily have taken the time off.

I called my wife and told her my decision, and she was surprised, but agreed for me to follow my instincts.

On September 2nd the Swissair disaster occurred on a plane leaving Kennedy airport in New York, which crashed in Newfoundland Canada with all lives lost.

I would not have originally been booked on that flight, but could have easily ended up on it since I was due to fly through Kennedy airport, and any delay might have caused me to switch planes.

I will never know for sure, but this was a very strong warning.

I should also mention that for several years before this event I had strong feelings that my I would be killed in the near future. After this happened those feelings ended.

c.   A few Seconds Ahead

Sometimes just having sensitivity about what will happen a few seconds into the future will have a positive effect.

Avoiding a car accident at an intersection is one result.

I believe animals have spiritual abilities too.

Here is an example concerning our last dog Apollo. Some years ago he was watching my wife as she planned to start disconnecting a motor inside our dishwasher.

Apollo started barking madly at us (which he never did) and we suddenly realized that we hadn't turned off the power to the dishwasher.

He seemed to be sensing a future event which made him really worried.

d.   Dreams of Indian Ocean Tsunami in 2004

Back around the year 2000 through 2004 I was having a series of dreams which were similar but all slightly different.

I seemed to be in a tropical coastal area and at some type of resort. There were lots of people on the beach and there were different types of resorts in each dream.

I had a lot of fear and then it happened. There would be some type of huge wave which crashed over us, or the tide would go out and a huge wave would come in and I would be covered by the wave.

When that happened I never escaped but seemed to be one of the victims.

I recall this type of dream happening at least five to ten times over that multi year period.

Of course the disaster finally happened—the late December 2004 Tsunami of the Indian Ocean which killed at least one quarter million persons.

Scientists researching this event now think this may have been the worst Tsunami disaster in over 600 years in the Indian Ocean.

I have since had a few dreams about Tsunamis hitting Southern California where I live, but none recently…

e.   Telepathy

In about 1995 my wife and I were at home and her teenage daughter Alex was visiting a Church across town with friends.

Suddenly the plate my wife was holding in the kitchen shattered in her hands.

She immediately felt that something had happened to Alex.

We had a call within a half hour and found out Alex had fallen at least 20 feet through a skylight. Fortunately, she only had minor injuries.

This type of sensitivity may have been simultaneous to the event, but it is also a good illustration of how persons with close emotional ties can sense dangerous events when or slightly before they are happening.

I also had an instance of waiting for a light to change at a busy intersection a few years ago.

When the light changed, for some reason I delayed going through even though I'm usually first through the intersection.

> A few seconds later a car from the cross street raced through the intersection and would certainly have hit my car if I hadn't delayed my crossing.

> This event shows that we can often have a time sense even just a few seconds into the future and it can be enough to save us from danger.

Chapter 10: What Prophets have in common

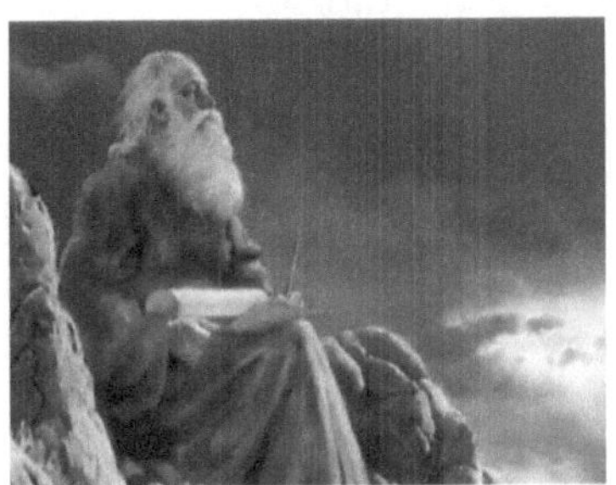

Figure 25-Depiction of a

True prophets have some traits in common which can be identified as enabling their abilities to provide some accuracy in predicting future events.

a.   Connection to God and Spirit

The most important of these traits is a person's spirituality. This means how close they are to the core of their being or spirit.

It should not be a surprise that many of the great religious leaders were also known as prophets. Those persons had spiritual authority with their people and the ability to prophesize just added more moral authority to their efforts.

As I'm emphasizing throughout this book, the ability to know your higher self which exists outside of time and space is a necessary requirement to having a real prophetic or pre-cognitive ability.

b.		Be willing to trust Intuition

It's not enough to just have visions or impressions of the future. A person needs to have some faith in what they are seeing and not dismiss it out of hand as an just "day dreaming" or as some type of hallucination.

You need to have confidence in your abilities. Confidence is usually gained over time as the individual sees that their predictions have some relation to what actually occurs.

c. A person grounded in Reality

A prophet has to be able to distinguish between what is really happening and what they think will happen.

They can't be successful in the long term if they are only having delusions which have no basis in fact or potential futures.

A real prophet will also have wisdom and use their abilities wisely to help build towards a goal, not just to impress people.

Chapter 11: Some Theories on how Prophecy works

a. The Nature of Reality

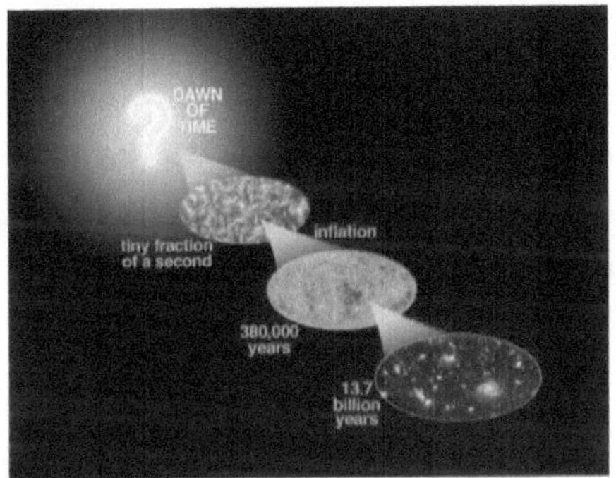

Figure 26-The Growth of the Universe

As I discussed in my book on immortality, I have some specific ideas on the nature of Reality and the core of our consciousness or spirit:

Physicists and Astronomers all agree that the Universe we know was created in a huge explosion called the "Big Bang". This was when the Universe was created from nothing and inflated. As it inflated time and space as we know them came into existence.

When you study Einstein's Relativistic Physics you being to understand that time and space are inextricably linked. You can't have one without the other.

Given our understanding of Physics, we know that time and space didn't exist before the Big Bang. The state of things before creation then was "No Time & No Space".

Another subject of great interest to Astrophysicists is what are called "Black Holes". Black Holes are a result of Einstein's equations and Astronomers have verified their existence in the last few decades.

Black Holes are stars which due to their own mass have collapsed down to an infinitely small point and where time stops. Scientists do not understand where all that mass goes.

Hmm…. A   Black Hole seems to be another example of part of reality that exists without time and space.

In Quantum Physics, time is also viewed differently that we perceive it on a daily basis. Here is a quote from a Physics website explaining this view: (17)

> *The upshot is that, on the microscopic level, there just plain is no direction to time -- and this is even more spectacularly true in quantum physics than in classical physics. In the microscopic domain, everything just exists in a kind of nebulous, atemporal continuum. Then, every once in a while, something becomes observable, and enters*

> *the one-dimensional time continuum. The arrow of time does not exist in the universe as a whole. It only exists in individual subjective views of the universe!*

I think it is fair to say that the place of stillness where time and space don't exist is a part of our reality.

Therefore, it shouldn't be considered too strange that our immortal Spirit is part of and one with that Stillness.

Given the above evidence of Science and my thinking I conclude that time is really an illusion of our physical being.

If we can pierce the illusion, we can expand our "time sense".

b. The Probability of the Future

One thing I have learned from my experiences is that the future is a probability, not a fixed event which is fated to happen.

However, as I learned from the Airplane ticket experience, it can be very difficult to change some futures.

I really had to put a lot of mental energy into fighting the desire to buy the plane ticket after being warned—because I really wanted to be with my family in Spain.
That's why I tried to buy the tickets three times.

I remember having to consciously fight my "need" to go and having to use very strong will power to overcome it since I knew that I had to follow my intuition since it was a very strong one.

I was even able to look forward and get a "feeling" that there would be a major crash on Sept 2nd.

Whereas with the Surfboard vision, I forgot all about it at the beach and it happened exactly as I saw it. I had intended to remember this vision since it was so strong, but when I got there my memory just disappeared.

There seems to be a certain momentum to the time stream and it takes a lot of effort to change it.

The analogy of a river of time is a good one. We normally flow with the current, but by force of will, we can change where we are in the stream, go upstream, and even go downstream.

c. The Yoga Sutras of Patanjali

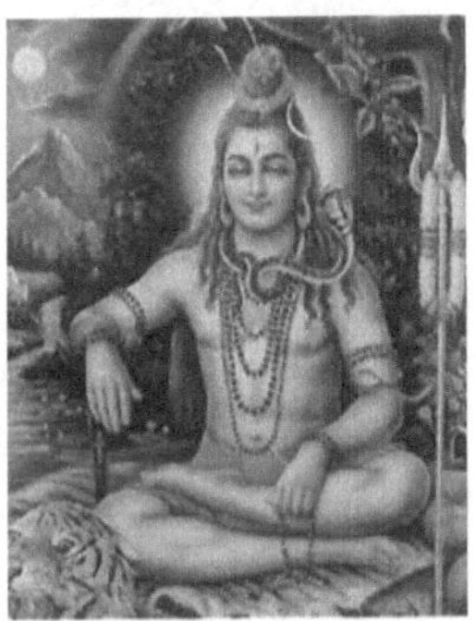

Figure 27-An artist's conception of Patanjali

Now for one of my favorite metaphysical books which was written in Sanskrit two thousand years ago "The Yoga Sutras of Patanjali". It was written as a scientific exposition on the path to enlightenment, and the abilities and spiritual states obtained as part of the process.

Book 3 Chapters 14 and 16 can be translated as follows:

14. Every object has its characteristics which are already quiescent,
those which are active, and those which are not yet definable.

The explanation is as follows:

Every object has characteristics belonging to its past, its present and its future.

In a fir tree, for example, there are the stumps or scars of dead branches, which once represented its foremost growth; there are the branches with their needles spread out to the air; there are the buds at the end of each branch and twig, which carry the still closely packed needles which are the promise of the future. In like manner, the chrysalis has, as its past, the caterpillar; as its future, the butterfly. The man has, in his past, the animal; in his future, the angel. Both are visible even now in his face. So with all things, for all things change and grow.

16. Through perfectly concentrated Meditation on the three stages of development comes a knowledge of past and future.

With an exposition on its meaning to be:

We have taken our illustrations from natural science, because, since every true discovery in natural science is a divination of a law in nature, attained through a flash of genius, such discoveries really represent acts of spiritual perception, acts of perception by the spiritual man, even though they are generally not so recognized. So we may once more use the same illustration. Perfectly concentrated Meditation, perfect insight into the chrysalis, reveals the caterpillar that it has been, the butterfly that it is destined to be. He who knows the seed, knows the seed-pod or ear it has come from, and the plant that is to come from it. So in like manner he who really knows today, and the heart of to-day, knows its parent yesterday and its child tomorrow.

Past, present and future are all in the Eternal. He who dwells in the Eternal knows all three.

When reviewing the Yoga Sutras we see that the ancient view of consciousness was that because it is rooted in the eternal.

Therefore, those who have developed themselves so that they perceive things from the point of view of the Spirit can sense the time states in all objects.

d.   More on the Illusion of Time

Below are excerpts from a dialog (18) between Andrew Cohen Swami Krishnananda. These two persons are widely recognized as being realized beings living in today's world, so their metaphysical perspective on time is a very useful viewpoint.

Swami Krishnananda (to Andrew Cohen): There are many people sitting here and they want to listen to you.

Andrew: So the message for today is: **dare to give up the illusion of time**. Give up the belief that there is any distance or gap between oneself and one's true Self, and between oneself and the rest of life, the rest of existence. This takes a lot of courage. It takes a willingness to die absolutely and unconditionally right now. So my message for today, and for every day, for every moment, is not to wait one second longer. That's my message.

K: So short! Please expand it with a little bit more detail.

A: Expand it? Okay. Well, many, many seekers believe with fervor and with great conviction that it will take them a very long time and much hard work to bridge the gap between where they are now and where they want to be. But it is this belief and conviction that there is this gap in the first place that creates the illusion of separation. Now if we have the courage to give up the illusion of separation, then we will find that we have no place to stand. And as we look and look we will not be able to locate ourselves. Everywhere we look we'll see nothing. We'll see nothing, and we'll see everything at the same time. So to come to this point, it takes great courage. Because if we want to know that much and see that much and be that much, we have to be willing to let go of every thought, notion or idea that we have about who we are, or about what's true. In order to do this we have to be willing to die unconditionally to the Absolute, and we have to be willing to give everything—and everything and everything and everything—to that and that alone; even our sadhana [spiritual practice], even that which we hold most precious and most dear to us. So that we're left empty and naked, and we have nothing and nothing and nothing at all.

K: You said one sentence that was very beautiful: we should remove the idea of the distance between what we are and what we ought to be.

A: Yes, time.

K: Does it exist? You are believing in a thing that does not exist. What makes you feel that time exists when you cannot see it anywhere? At least space you can see, there is a vast expanse. But have you seen time? Yet time conditions the whole world. "Your destiny is in the hands of time," as they say. How could you accept such a thing called time which cannot be seen with the eyes. How is it that it cannot be seen? The reason for this also must be known. An existent thing must be seen. People say, "There is no proof that God exists, because he can't be seen with any available means of experiment or perception." But have you seen time? And yet you believe in time.

Imagine that you were going to be executed tomorrow. What will you be thinking in your mind today? Your soul will tremble and nobody knows what it will do. Tomorrow you will know.

When you are drowning and there is no hope of survival, the true self comes up and sees what can be done. When you have lost everything and nobody wants to look at your face, you will develop a great strength.

K: Will anybody believe? **There is a whole world of illusion, maya, as they call it**. Is it true that tomorrow we shall realize the truth?

A: This is the greatest challenge I think for the true seeker: to give up time, to give up the future.

K: There is no such thing as the future. When time is gone, the future also goes. There is eternity. In eternity there is no yesterday and tomorrow, it is just here. And if you believe that God exists and God is eternity, it is impossible to conceive what the state of affairs is. The supreme Absolute is dancing in our hearts and we are closing our eyes to that dance.

The sentences I've highlighted in bold are key to the enlightened understanding that time is an illusion. If we can look at this illusion from our spirits then the whole of past, present, and future becomes visible since the spirit lives outside of time and space.

Chapter 12: Exercises to Awaken your Prophetic Abilities

I'll start this chapter on awakening with some of my own techniques to see the future.

a. Learning to Meditate or Pray Deeply

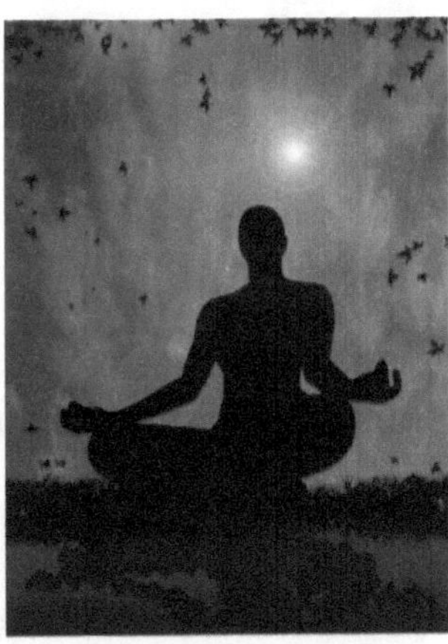

Figure 28-A Person

First, it is key to be able to get in touch with your spirit, and the best way to do that is through learning meditation or deep prayer techniques.

Meditation is the key to developing most spiritual abilities since it allows one to calm down the mind and start to perceive your higher self or spirit. It is this spirit

In Appendix A at the end of this book I've listed some of my instructions on learning to meditate.

There are also a couple of books in the Bibliography on techniques to meditate.

Meditation is best learned through an instructor. These days there are many instructors to choose from in the major cities.

b. Visualizing the Future

Once you are in a very relaxed state your consciousness will not be distracted.

The next thing to do is to start visualizing yourself in a future scene as accurately as possible.

When I had the vision described earlier in this book about the surfboard accident I was meditating deeply. While meditating I was going through my mind about places I intended to visit on the vacation trip I was planning later in the summer. While thinking about the beach on Cape Cod and what I might do there like surfing was when I had the vision.

I must have tuned into a major probable event in my life because then I was just there and saw the scene exactly as it later happened—from the viewpoint of being in my own body and the accident happening to me.

c. Checking the Future for Problems

One of the habits I've acquired in my life is to look ahead before I take a trip somewhere. I do it so often it has become a habit.

When I had the warnings of danger about buying plane tickets to Spain, I was thinking about the upcoming trip, the flight over there, and what I would do there.

The Danger warning I received came as kind of a "dark cloud of death" that gave me a lot of fear whenever I started thinking about buying the plane tickets. I have never had a reaction like that before or since when planning to buy travel tickets.

Another story illustrates what happens when you don't follow your intuition or haven't defined it in detail.

We were planning a family trip to Disneyworld for the Spring of 2008. Prior to the trip I did my usual review of what we would be doing. For some reason I had the impression of a black border around Epcot--not a deep dark fatal feeling. Just the feeling that something would go wrong that would be a personal problem.

I should have delved deeper into the things we might do there. Maybe I would have gotten a more specific warning-and saved myself a very uncomfortable day.

When we were there I agreed to take the "Orange Ticket" ride on the Space Ride and became very motion sick. Then I threw up on the ride and had to go to the infirmary for several hours.

This was a situation that could have been avoided if I'd had just a little more forethought and review of the planned activities there.

d. Harold Sherman's Insights

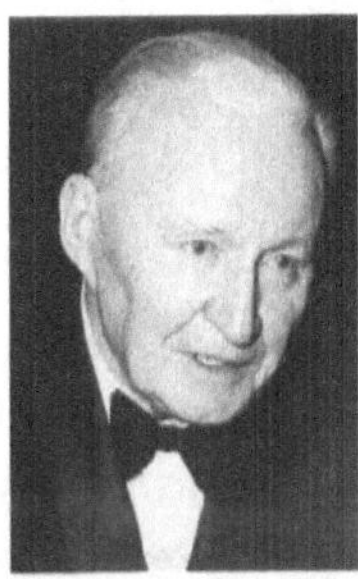

Figure 29-Picture of Harold Sherman -Psychic and Writer

Harold Sherman was born July 13, 1898 in Traverse City, Michigan and died in 1987.

He was a powerful psychic and wrote many books on the paranormal.

His ideas on foreseeing the future are very similar to the ones I've developed over the years.

In the Chapter in his book called "How to Foresee and Control your Future" (19) on seeing the future of others he states the following:

> "The technique for sensing what is going to happen to others is to relax, physically and mentally, and to place yourself in *feeling attunement* with them.
>
> (By this he means to think of them and what the person is about and imagine you are in their head and thinking their thoughts)

Let yourself wonder, sincerely and sympathetically, what you can do to help them. This is the sole reason why you want to concern yourself with their future. Don't try to impose yourself upon their private lives or to determine knowledge of their innermost thoughts, aspirations, intentions, god or bad for your own personal gain.

If you seek to use your higher powers of mind in this way, to try to influence others for your own selfish purposes, you may get the wrong impressions and arouse mental as well as physical resistance.

Give the right, receptive attitude of mind motivated by love, you will be amazed at how easily and quietly you suddenly know what future prospects of others are, and what your own future can be or may be, with relation to them."

With regard to controlling your own future some excerpts are as follows:

"Yes-It is important to keep the mental image of what you want to do or be or have in consciousness. See it in your mind's eye as though it has already happened. Let the creative power take you from where you are, step by step, to where you want to be. As you fill in part of the picture by actual developments or achievements, concentrate on the parts you have not yet brought into being….Just KNOW that as you continue to put forth earnest sincere efforts towards your goal, that this Higher Power within will be working right along with you".

It also helps to act out what you are picturing. Harold tells this story:

A an article in the editorial section of the Little Rock Gazette for May 26, 1968 regarding the Prime Minister of England Harold Wilson

"When Wilson was a boy of ten—42 years ago—he told his parents his ambition was to be Prime Minister. He posed in cloth cap and short trousers in front of 10 Downing Street, London, the minister's residence. His election fulfilled the dream."

e. Learning to Predict Major and World Happenings

There is a vibrational frequency that we can all attune to when looking for what future events may hold.

One technique to focus your perception of future events follows:

- Get into a relaxed meditate state to calm down your thoughts and emotions
- While holding your mind in stillness ask yourself a question like "What is going to happen to me with relation to some situation in which I'm interested or involved.
- Write down your impressions
- Reach down into your mind and tell your subconscious to seek a more specific answer to this query.

An example might be to ask yourself "Is there going to be another large hurricane in New Orleans?" Then wait for impressions in that relaxed state and write them down.

You may need to repeat this activity several times to make sure you aren't just living your fears or desires.

The objective of this exercise is to connect with your spirit's insight—for your perception to not be muddied by our daily fears, concerns or desires.

Chapter 13: Using Prophecy in your life

a. Avoiding Accidents

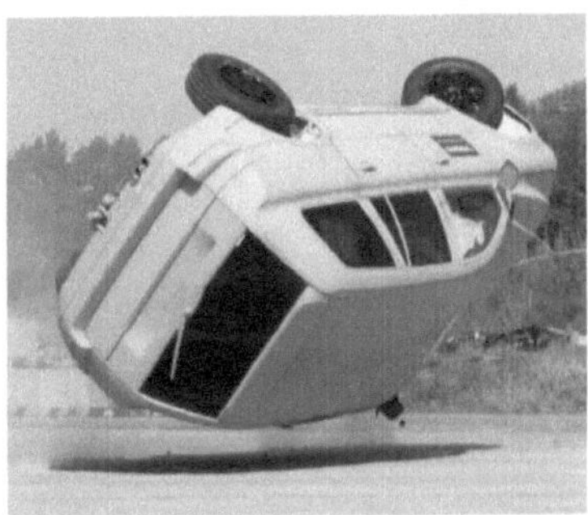

Figure 30-Picture of an accident

One of the most common ways to use your precognitive abilities are to keep yourself out of danger.

As the numerous examples in this book demonstrate, my life has been saved numerous times by my future time sense.

Making future review of upcoming events a habit in your daily life will pay off big dividends at some point

I always try to imagine myself taking the trip I'm planning, or visualizing how a certain event or activity will go. Not always, but often I get ideas about those events to better plan ahead. Sometimes I also get a warning to not attend or do the activity.

Appendix B contains a list of situations/accidents/potential accidents I survived. They are ranked by

A—Accidents/Potentials which would surely have killed me.
B—Accidents which could likely have killed
C—Accidents which might have killed me

The ability to avoid accidents is a learned one.

Part of the Spiritual development process can be to expand your "time sense" to detect danger before it happens. This can be from a few seconds before a car goes through and intersection to weeks, months, or years involving major life events.

In my own life I've experienced numerous times where I was saved by some "Spiritual Force" from a major accident or death.

Some of my accident avoidance experience clearly had a paranormal or spiritual component.

The one that comes to mind the most is #10 in the table in Appendix B.—my "almost mugged" experience. I would have definitely walked right into the muggers if my body hadn't sent me this urgent signal that I had to urinate. I just couldn't go forward. When I tried twice I was stopped each time. Then the muggers came out from behind pillars and started walking towards us. This was when my friend and I took off running and got away.

Learning to use your spiritual senses to avoid trouble and accidents will become more important the older you get.

If you ever have an intuition of "danger" or "something is not right" I suggest you follow it.

Some persons experience pre-cognitive dreams where they dream of a terrible event happening to them or others. Later the event does happen. I remember a few years ago I had five or more dreams over months about different tropical beach resorts. Then the water all receded and later came in as a huge wave.

This was all prior to the Indian Ocean Tsunami. The dreams stopped after the event.

Since the future is only a potential, you can make, and persons have made decisions to allow them to avoid the accident they saw and therefore change their own future.

b. Controlling your Future

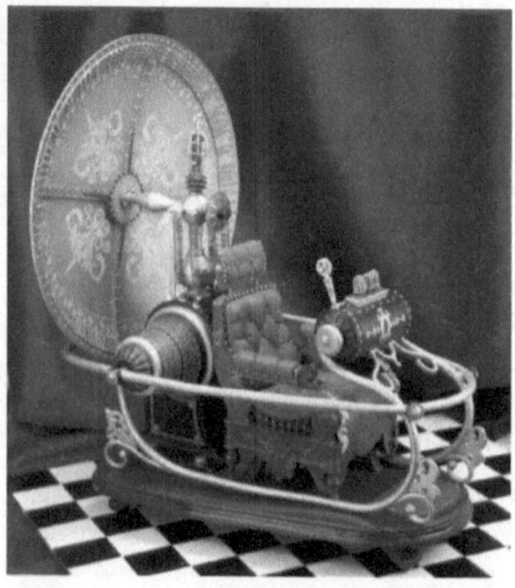

Figure 31-An Artist's rendering of a Time Machine

One of the things you can do with an increased time sense is to actually control your future.

Since the future is a probability, you can affect it in most cases.

I say most cases because there are some world shaking events like major disasters or wars where the "energy" involved in those events is much greater than any one individual is likely to be able to modify.

Here is another example from my life:

I decided a few years ago to build a fallout shelter into the hillside in my backyard.

I kept visualizing it every day as a completed structure. Imagining the design, the walls, how it would be stocked, etc.

As I kept visualizing it my mind poured "energy" into it.

After a couple of weeks of this effort one day it just seemed to me that the "Thought Form" I had created was complete. That the structure would be there and there was no need for further work on it mentally.

The resources and materials did come together and the shelter was finished very quickly.

Now you can be skeptical about this experience, but many writers on the paranormal will testify to the effect of thought forms on events that will happen.

One of the best books I've read on this subject is Thought-forms by Annie Besant and C.W. Leadbeater.

According to them, "Thought Forms" are created by all minds. Some thoughts re-inforce each other, while some are specific to different persons.

The idea here is that the thoughts you have created with your mind have an effect on the future. Your thoughts become the "blueprint" for what will happen—good or bad.

This is not a book on Thought forms but I strongly believe in our thought's abilities to affect the future.

From a metaphysical perspective, the world we see is an illusion. Much of it is generated out of the collective unconscious of our minds.

Our minds provide the energy and the pattern for the future.

Therefore, our individual thoughts have a major impact on the future.

Doing conscious visualization of the result we would like in some future event will have an effect on that event occurring.

Again, if the event is a major one our individual impact may be minor.

One of Jesus's quotes from the Bible is relevant here:

> Luke 17:5-6 "The apostles said to the Lord, 'Increase our faith!' The Lord replied. 'If you had faith the size of a mustard seed, you could say to this mulberry tree, 'Be uprooted and planted in the sea,' and it would obey you.'"

To have this effect one needs to visualize the outcome already exists—not how to get there.

In other words if you plan to win a baseball game then imagine you have already won it and visualize the scene as clearly as possible. The more times you do it before the event the better.

This whole approach goes along with the concepts that the future is malleable and can change. Also, that in many real ways, the future is an illusion which the mind controls.

Chapter 14: Using Prophecy with Wisdom

What does wisdom have to do with Prophecy you may ask?

First of all, I believe that if one is gifted enough to have or be able to develop the ability to foretell the future, then you have a moral and ethical duty to use this ability for good and productive uses to help our fellow man.

Also, since the future is not fixed, our actions can affect the future for good or ill.

A person who has relatively accurate predictions will gain a lot of credibility with others. This influence can be used constructively, or for selfish gain.

The ability to tell the future is after all based on a connection to one's spirit.

Being able to help others with their spiritual development should always be a goal for a person who influences others through their predictions.

The ability to do Prophecy is a side effect ability of spiritual development—not an end in itself.

This is something to keep in the forefront of you mind as you become more involved in prophecies, predictions, or divination.

May you be blessed in your future spiritual evolution and use these abilities in a productive and helpful way on your journey.

An Exercise in Avoiding Accidents

(Video Transcription)

So the biggest danger once you've reached a stable long-term health is how do you avoid accidents? New anecdotal evidence is that a lot of immortals have learned to avoid danger in accidents.

I will tell you in my life when I was writing my immortality book I compiled a list of 27 events that I've been through-some of which were major, and some more minor, which could have killed me. Some of which I definitely avoided because I was able to use my time sense. I have a very good time sense. If I have any ability that I was born with is my natural ability on prophecies. I'm very strong in prophecy.

I've had a lot of things happen to me in this life both for major events and personal events in my life and sometimes other people and so I've learned from that. And I've learned how to utilize premonitions in my life. And there's a lot of techniques to sense danger and also sense good events in the future.

Remember if we believe that the spirit which is the core of our being-lives outside of time and space. It has an oversight of time space, and so part of us has an ability to ride the time stream-to see outside of the now, and see what's potentially coming up in the future. Now when we talk about the future, the future is a probability the future which hasn't happened yet. There are ways to look at the future and see the probability of certain events occurring. Some events have a lot of energy in those probabilities and they're almost certain to occur because of the energy some can be changed. And I can tell you that there's a lot of momentum for certain probabilities to happen, for certain events to happen, and that you can override them-but it's not easy. It depends on the event so there's multiple potential futures and we can decide what future we want-to go down the path we want to go down. This has to do with a certain visualization technique and force of will.

One of the good books I recall reading on this which first introduced me to a lot of this, was a book by Harold Sherman back in the 1970s. Titled "How to Foresee and Control your Future". He had a lot of good techniques that he thought about. Okay-so I'm going to talk about some of my personal examples that led me to my current understanding about how this all works, and how we can use it in avoiding accidents.

The first major event I had in my life of this type was when i was in about nineteen seventy-five. I was a co-op summer engineering employee at General Electric gas turbine engineering in New York State, and I was meditating during the lunch of time. I was kind of the young hippie engineer according to these old guys so they let me alone. I thought I was weird, but they let me do it so I was sitting at my desk meditating during the lunch period and I was going to leave a couple weeks. I was going to take a trip to Cape Cod. I want to drive out to Cape Cod see what's going on, so while I'm meditating I'm thinking about my trip to Cape Cod and I'm kind of mentally going through what I was going to do out there. The places i might want to stay, and the things I might want to do, and all of a sudden I had this incredible vision-I mean it was a brilliant realistic vision during day time when I was not dreaming but just in the deep state-and what I saw is I was a surfboard trying to surf because I hadn't learned how to do it. Then a big wave hit me I fell off I came up from under the water and the thing went BAM it threw me out in a meditation. I just like woke up and I thought wow that was too real. What happened here? So I kind of didn't think too much about it and a couple weeks later I was out on Cape Cod walking around the beach and there were some guys with some surfboards. I said hey "where can I rent one" and they said "we've got some extra ones. Do you want to you want to try with us?" So I said sure of course forgetting my whole dream at the time. So I went out there to try and surf and I'm not I'm not very good at all-trying to get up on that thing is not easy. So I spent all day trying to get up when I got up a little bit and would fall off, and about two in the afternoon I'm getting pretty exhausted. I try it again and the same scene exactly happens. I fall off from the wave, go under, come up and then the board hits me BAM in my chin. A terrible hit-I was all bloody. I staggered out of the water they took me to the hospital. I had like ten stitches and two sutures in my chin and I think my jaw was broken too.

Okay, so I was not feeling good about that but I thought wow this is really amazing. Something I foresaw a couple weeks ago actually happened to me. Okay so that was the first time I didn't avoid that at all-but it led me to understand that those things were real. That people could really see an event happening in their future a few years later. And this is a little different because I've had lots of different ways of these things coming to me they're not all an incredible visualization. Some are much different.

For instance, a few years later I graduated from college, and I was driving through Detroit where a friend of mine lived. I stopped to see him and we went to this place which I think is now the headquarters of General Motors which was a set of buildings in in downtown Detroit which had been built in a slum—The Renaissance Center. We ate dinner there, and understand this is in the late 1970s and the lower area of it was all boarded up because there just weren't any stores to open up there. So my friend Steve and I are walking out on the lower level after we've eaten dinner and we're in an area that's totally deserted. There's nobody but us and I'd say we're about as far from just beyond that door there-there's a pillar and I suddenly stopped I had this incredible urge-I had to go to the bathroom. Steve said "Why are you stopping?". I don't know-I suddenly have this big urge to go to the bathroom. Bathrooms are back the other way. I tried to go forward again and I had to stop again I could not go forward. I just had I had this incredible thing I had to go as soon as possible and as soon as that happened the second time-out from behind the pillar these two black guys wearing trench coats came out and they started walking towards us We could not tell I didn't know what they had under their trench coats. They might have guns, so they looked at me they looked at us, and my friend Steve took off running. We were big young guys, but we figured we don't know what type of weapons they've got. And I thought about it a second, so I took off running also. They took off chasing us and we got back into the area where everyone was. There was a policeman, so they just kind of smiled-next time we will get you. They left us alone. So I got a warning. I didn't expect that warning. I don't know if it was an angel watching me, or something of my consciousness seeing this time stream, but I got this incredible warning which saved my life.

There was another event about a plane flight. Okay some of you have heard this story but I'll tell it again. Back in 1998-I was married at the time-my family we'd all made a decision to take a trip to Barcelona, because my wife's mother lived in Barcelona, and we wanted to see her. We wanted to have a good time. My stepdaughter at the time and my son who was only a year old went with my wife. I was also trying to get this big project to work on as a contractor at Boeing, and I'd been waiting for it for like a month or two but it hadn't closed yet so there was enough going on I was talking to enough people on the phone that I figured maybe I should wait a while and not go over there yet. So I told my wife to go ahead and I'd come over a week or two later after things were settled. So they went ahead and I didn't really like to do that but I figured I needed to do that so I could try and establish some income. So they get over there and about a week I'm trying to make a decision about going. Realized I'm just wasting my time here. I can put the dog in the kennel because I really wanted to be with my family. Okay so I decided to try and call the travel agency to get some tickets. Now I try to make the call-I try to pick up the phone, and call a travel agency, and then I got this really dark black feeling. I put the phone down.

I didn't do anything-that's weird, so I tried later in the day. I tried to call a travel agency again. I pick up the phone again I call again, and I get a really dark black feeling like don't do this. It's hard to explain. I put the phone down again. The next day I'm really pushing and I call a travel agency. I get somebody on the line and I get the same feeling again. I had to hang up and I thought oh my god-if I go on this flight something really bad is going to happen to me. It was like a real deep feeling so I thought about it and I thought about the previous experiences I had and it was more than just the ones I mentioned. I thought if I've learned anything I've learned I need to pay attention when i get these types of signals and I really wanted to go.

I had a lot of emotional energy invested in going so I really thought about it for hours and I meditated on it. I sat down to use the technique that I'm going to teach you to look forward-look at the next couple of weeks-look at when I thought I was going to go over there which was September second. I had this image of a plane crash. A big plane crash and I thought this is not right. There's something wrong here. I should also mention that for the previous couple of years leading up to this I'd had this feeling that I was going to die-I mean some people say they get these feelings when their life is going to end. I had this feeling my time was coming up. So all these things were together and it was a really tough decision because you really want to be with your family. You really want to go do something. You may lose the opportunity, versus some stupid fear that you've got about the upcoming events. I did I made the decision-which was tough-because again we're talking about the momentum of an event that you're moving towards. I called my wife and I said to her "look I just had this really bad feeling" and I told her what had happened and she had some understanding of things that happened to me. She had some events in her life like this so she said okay if you really feel you need to do that. So we said fine and I stayed home. And I felt pretty stupid for a couple weeks.

September second 1998 the Swiss Air flight crashed in the Ocean in Newfoundland, Canada, and killed 150 people. That was likely a flight I would have been on. I can't ever say for sure it would have been, but I had very high probability being a flight that would have been my death.

This is one of those events you can't prove that it would have happened but I think I avoided it and after that time my I feel my long-term feelings that had for the previous two years about my time being up went away-it was gone. I felt like I had a totally new lease on life and I've never had that type of event happen since then. So that was a major thing for me that I actually thought I had changed the probability of my own future.

All right, a little lighter story back four or five years ago. We took a family trip to Disney World. We going to visit there and we're visiting the different centers. I'm doing my visualization of the trip in my mind ahead of time and I I'm looking in my mind at Epcot and I'm kind of seeing a dotted black line around it. I'm thinking what's going on here? I thought am I going to die? And Epcot gave me the impression-no I'm not going to die but something bad may will happen. So I kind of put it out of my mind we went on the trip. The trip looked reasonable.

I knew it was going be okay till we got there, and we do the things we planned. We ended up at Epcot one day and my son says "You want to go on the Mars ride?" I said "Sure". He said "You want the orange sticker or the green ticket?" He said what's the difference was that with the orange tickets they spin you around. I was being adventurous so I said "Sure let's go on the orange ticket ride". So we stood in line to get in the orange ticket ride. I thought after looking at it-that is not such a good idea. So we get in and this thing starts spinning and I lose it. I throw up all over the console, and I throw up all over myself, and my wife, and we get out of this ride. I staggered over to this little cleanup room that they have just for people like me and I clean up my shirt and I get out of there. Then I go over and I lie down the infirmary for like two hours. I'm just lying in the infirmary so I think that's what my senses were trying to tell me-That I was going to live but I might not have a good time. That's right.

So I'll just tell you one other story which is not along these lines-it's more of a general nature-and then we'll get into doing the exercise. But, I had these dreams back before two thousand and four for the previous couple of years, where I would be in these resorts with palm trees. They would be different resorts, and I'd be enjoying myself, and then the ocean would go out and this huge tidal wave would come in. And I didn't know why I had so many dreams-I must have had 10 dreams about this and I'm wondering why I got this fixation with tsunamis overwhelming resorts. And then of course the Indian Ocean tsunami happened and my dreams became true. So i don't know I had that happen, but that made an impact on me too.

So any questions so far before we get into the exercise? Alright, so to do this you want to get into that relaxed state again. So why don't you do that everybody for a couple of minutes here and then we'll start the exercise. I'll sit down here. As you are closing you're closing your eyes, and getting relaxed, what I want you to do, is I want you to pick a trip you plan to make or event you plan to attend within the next year.

It could be a simple trip, it could be a trip to visit a friend, or relative, or could be some events you've been planning. It could even be just be a birthday party. It doesn't have to be any complex or extensive thing ok-this is the event we're going to look at the future context about. Now we're going to start imagining that we're on a trip to that event and for instance what is going on if it's a plane flight. Imagine we're going through this, we're in the terminal, we're boarding the plane, or it could be just getting in a car. We're on the transportation now, we're feeling how it looks, how it feels-the temperature, the color, like we're really there.

While we're doing this I want you to keep thinking, I want you to get impressions emotionally: Do I feel safe, do I feel unsafe, happy, sad? What we're going to do is draw emotions out of the continuum about our event. So we're traveling to the event now-we're going to reach our destination. We get off a plane or get out of the car or off the train. We get to our destination. We're doing the activities we want to do there, whether it's walking around, or talking to our friends. We're feeling-how do you feel now? Do you feel happy, do you feel sad? Do you feel worried? Do you feel any blackness or do you feel any light?

Keep remembering these impressions because we're going to go through this little exercise a second time. Okay- now the event is completing, now we're leaving the event. We're coming back through the transportation. How does everything look? How's the weather? Is it day or night? Are we with other people or by ourselves? And what is our state of mind? Are we feeling good?

Now that the event is over we're back where we started. We're not done though, now we're going to go through this whole scenario again. Same event, same bar, same destination, and we've done it once, now we're going to visualize it more fully. Okay-so now we're starting off again. We're going to the destination, we're imagining our surroundings. The weather day or night, people, animals, the smells, the feelings, how motions feel, what are our senses. Is picking up good or bad? Now we're getting to the event, or at the event, things are going on, the activities you wanted to do, to people you want to talk to. The things you were going to buy, whatever that is again since is it good or bad good feeling. Bad feelings are danger. See if you notice any similar points to your last trip through this, because we're trying to find consistent feelings about this event. Now the event is finished. Now we're leaving, coming back everything, that's going on again in your five senses. What does all feel like? And your emotions-how do you feel emotionally? Did things work out well? Did you have an argument with somebody? Did you fall in love with somebody? Any emotions that you can feel, and also was it consistent with something that happened the first time around?

Okay-take a minute to just slowly come out of it. I know we did that probably fairly quickly. But I would like to know if anybody got any impressions there. Any impressions about your event?- good? Bad? Was it a success? Is their problem okay the second time when we went there?

I found this very useful if you practice this. And I do it now for all my events. I just don't even take a long time. I take half a minute before I go somewhere and I found it's amazingly effective. I think it will work for everyone once you get to feeling that you can see forward in your time sense, and I think we all can. It's just being open to the impressions and following your intuition. When you get a serious impression. So I wanted to share that because I thought it's important to the whole subject we're doing this weekend.

Articles on Prophecy Techniques

Palm Reading

1. Choose a hand. For females, the right hand is what you're born with, and left is what you've accumulated throughout your life. For males, it is the other way around. For male, the left hand is what you're born with, and right is what you've accumulated throughout your life. But it can also be whichever hand is dominant, which can be your present/past life hand and the least dominant hand could be your future life hand. Pick a palm to read.

2. Identify the four major lines.
Identify the four major lines. (1) The heart line. (2) The head line. (3) The life line. (4) The fate line (Not everybody has this.)

3. Interpret the heart line. This line can be read in either direction (from the pinkie finger to the index finger or vice versa) depending on the tradition being followed.

It's believed to indicate emotional stability, romantic perspectives, depression, and cardiac health.

- Begins below the index finger - content with love life
- Begins below the middle finger - selfish when it comes to love
- Begins in the middle - falls in love easily.
- Straight and short - less interest in romance
- Touches life line - heart broken easily
- Long and curvy - freely expresses emotions and feelings
- Straight and parallel to the head line - good handle on emotions
- Wavy - many relationships and lovers, absence of serious relationships
- Circle on the line - sad or depression
- Broken line - emotional trauma
- Smaller lines crossing through heart line - emotional trauma

4. Examine the head line. Represents learning style, communication style, intellectualism, and thirst for knowledge. A curved line is associated with creativity and spontaneity, while a straight line is linked with practicality and a structured approach.

- Short line - prefers physical achievements over mental ones
- Curved, sloping line - creativity
- Separated from life line - adventure, enthusiasm for life.
- Wavy line - short attention span
- Deep, long line - thinking is clear and focused
- Straight line - thinks realistically

- o Donuts or cross in head line - emotional crisis
- o Broken head line - inconsistencies in thought
- o Multiple crosses through head line - momentous decisions

5. Evaluate the life line. Begins near the thumb and travels in an arc towards the wrist. Reflects physical health, general well being, and major life changes (e.g. cataclysmic events, physical injuries, and relocations). Its length is not associated with length of life.

- o Runs close to thumb - often tired
- o Curvy - plenty of energy
- o Long, deep - vitality.
- o Short and shallow - manipulated by others
- o Swoops around in a semicircle - strength and enthusiasm.
- o Straight and close to the edge of the palm - cautious when it comes to relationships
- o Multiple life lines - extra vitality
- o Circle in line indicates - hospitalized or injured

o Break - sudden change in lifestyle

6. Study the fate line. This is also known as the line of destiny, and it indicates the degree to which a person's life is affected by external circumstances beyond their control. Begins at the base of the palm:

o Deep line - strongly controlled by fate
o Breaks and changes of direction - prone to many changes in life from external forces
o Starts joined to life line - self-made individual; develops aspirations early on
o Joins with the life line somewhere in the middle - signifies a point at which one's interests must be surrendered to those of others
o Starts at base of thumb and crosses life line - support offered by family and friends

7. Determine the hand shape. Each hand shape is associated with certain character traits. The length of the palm is measured from the wrist to the bottom of the fingers.

o Earth - broad, square palms and fingers, thick or coarse skin, and ruddy color; length of the palm equals length of fingers

- Solid values and energy, sometimes stubborn
- Practical and responsible, sometimes materialistic
- Work with their hands, comfortable with the tangible

- Air - square or rectangular palms with long fingers and sometimes protruding knuckles, low-set thumbs,

and dry skin; length of the palm less than length of
fingers
- Sociable, talkative and witty
- Can be shallow, spiteful and cold
- Comfortable with the mental and the intangible
- Does things in different and radical ways

o Water - long, sometimes oval-shaped palm, with long,
flexible, conical fingers; length of the palm equals length
of fingers but is less than width across the widest part of
the palm

- Creative, perceptive and sympathetic
- Can be moody, emotional and inhibited
- Introverts
- Do things quietly and intuitively.

o Fire - square or rectangular palm, flushed or pink skin,
and shorter fingers; length of the palm is greater than
length of fingers

- Spontaneous, enthusiastic and optimistic
- Sometimes egoistic, impulsive and insensitive
- Extroverts
- Do things boldly and instinctively

8. Palm reading is an awesome thing to do and I hope
you will try it!

Tips

- Try practicing on your own hands.
- Know that palm reading is not always accurate and
  that the fate of your life and your decisions should not
  be influenced by these things.

- In general, the more flexible the hand, the more flexible the person.
- Make sure the lighting in the area you are planning to read palms is good, for trying to do it in the dark makes it difficult to get a good read.
- Since palm lines change as you progress through life, palm reading is seen by many as an opportunity to reveal what's already happened, but not as a way of predicting the future.
- Note the texture of the hand, front and back. Soft hands signify sensitivity and refinement, while rough hands signifies a coarse temperament.
- Write down a chart for the 4 main lines (life, fate, heart, head) and hand types (fire, earth, air & water) do when you are just beginning to read palms you won't have to remember everything. Also, if you want to get good at it quick study the chart and you'll have it down in no time.

Simple Steps to Performing a Tarot Reading
by Bonnie Cehovet

The Tarot is one of the oldest divination oracles still in use today. It can be used in many ways, including meditation, visualization, and ritual work, but its widest use is in performing Tarot readings. The archetypes that make up the Tarot lend themselves to acting as a gateway between our conscious and unconscious selves, enabling us to connect with ancestral voices (and universal knowledge).

There are many different reasons for wanting to do a reading: to better understand the past; to bring the present into sharper focus; to see what our current options are; to see what the effect of taking a given action (or actions) will be on our life; as a tool for spiritual growth; as a tool for both mental and physical healing; as a tool for understanding/healing our relationships; as a tool to help us guide our careers - these are just a few of the myriad reasons for doing a reading.

So you sit down with your deck of choice. You may or may not have an idea of what you want to read for, or how you want to phrase your question. You may be at a loss as to which spread you want to work with, and you may truly be at a loss as to how to best interpret the spread once it is laid out. Time to take a deep breath, and exhale slowly. There is magick in the Tarot, but the key to unlocking that magick lies within the reader. Every reader needs to be open to allowing information to come through to them. Do not be afraid of what you see - you may see some shadows, but we all have them. They are a part of every reading that has ever been done.

Let's start our reading by defining the question/issue at hand. That is all we are going to think about right now. If you are reading for someone else, ask them to take some time, and think about what they want to ask. If, in the end, the question is open ended (i.e. along the lines of "What do I need to know about?), then form the question in exactly that manner. The answers that we receive are only as good as the questions that we ask. We want to state the question (which acts as the foundation for the reading) in as succinct a manner as possible. In other words - it should be brief, and to the point.

Note: As readers, we also need to make it clear to our clients that questions about finances, health, or legal advice are best left to professionals in those fields. Then there is the issue of "third party" questions. "Third parties" can be defined as anyone who is not present during a reading. My personal point of view is that if my client has a direct relationship with the party they are asking about, I will read for them. But I place definite boundaries here - I will read only in the areas that affect both people. If a client asks about a significant other, for instance, I will read for that. But I will not read for the significant other and someone else in the significant other's life, nor will I read for areas in the significant other's life that do not directly affect my client. I firmly believe in sacred space (personal boundaries), and feel that we should not cross these boundaries.

If you decide to read for yourself, try to be as objective as possible. Pretending that you are reading for someone else may help here. Your own emotions, if they enter too far into a reading, will essentially negate it.

I have found that questions are best expressed in the form of "What", rather than "Why". "What is the lesson that I need to learn?" will elicit a deeper response than "Why did this happen?" If you (or your client, if you are reading for someone else) know the general issue that you want to address, but are having a hard time formulating a specific question, take a few minutes and write down all of the questions that you might have. Go over these questions, define what is similar about them, and form a question that is relatively inclusive. For instance, if all of the questions are formed around career, a good question to ask might be: "What do I need to know about my work environment, and what actions will allow me to feel in greater control?"

Once the question has been defined (and don't be afraid to help your client reformat their question into something that will bring them a more inclusive, deeper answer), repeat it back to your client. Ask your client to hold the question in their mind as they shuffle the deck (or as you shuffle it, if that is your choice). (Note: If you choose to read with reversals, make sure that a certain percentage of the cards are reversed before they are shuffled for the reading.) It is this focus that will allow the Tarot to bring through the most in depth answers. A lack of focus at this point will result in a reading that may make little or no sense at all.

Note: At this pointing time, I silently ask my guides, and the guides of my client, to be with us during the reading. I ask that the information that is about to be brought through be of the highest quality, and that it bring clarity to my client.

Once the client is done shuffling, I ask them to take the deck in their left hand, and break it down into three piles, left to right. I then pick the cards up, placing the center pile over the pile on the left, and the combined pile on top of the pile to the right. There is no hard and fast rule here - this is just what I do. It is actually not necessary to do this at all.

Before laying out the cards, one more decision needs to be made. Some spreads have a built in significator (a card drawn to represent the Seeker), and some do not. I have never felt the need to read with a significator, and simply do not draw for that position when it is built into a spread that I am using. There is not hard and fast rule about this - it really comes down to what the reader is comfortable with.

If you decide to read with a significator, there are various ways that the card can be chosen. A card can be drawn at random, you can use your client's Zodiac sign to determine the suit (Wands are Aries, Leo is Sagittarius; Cups are Cancer, Scorpio, and Pisces; Swords are Gemini, Libra and Aquarius; Pentacles are Taurus, Virgo, and Capricorn), or you can use physical characteristics.

In the method using Zodiac signs, once the suit has been defined, the Court Card that best matches your client is chosen. Pages are most often seen as children (or teens) of either sex, Knights as young adults of either sex; Queens as adult females (or married women); and Kings as adult males (or married men). In the method using physical characteristics, the traditional view is: Wands are fair, with light or reddish hair and either light or dark eyes. Cups are fair, with light brown or dark blond hair, and gray, blue, or hazel eyes. Swords are olive complected, with brown or black hair, and light eyes. Pentacles are dark skinned, with black or dark brown hair, and dark eyes. Use the same system as above for determining which card within the suit best defines your client.

A more complicated method is the Myers-Briggs method, which works with personality types. Excellent references for this method are: Understanding The Tarot Court, by Mary K. Greer and Tom Little (Llewellyn Worldwide, 2005) and the Internet resource on Myers-Briggs..

As a reader, you are now going to lay down the cards in some type of format, and interpret them. You can choose to use a formal spread here, or you can read the cards at random. In either case, you need to keep the question in mind as you do the reading. In reading the cards at random, the technique of "free association" comes into play. The colors, and the images, within the card determine the meaning of the card, and the context that it is read in. In "Haindl Tarot - A Reader's Handbook" (U.S. Games Systems Inc., 1995), author Rachel Pollack states that for her, the best use for this type of reading is when she is reading for herself, or at the end of a more formal reading. It is also a technique that works well for psychic readers.

In most instances, a formal spread will be used. This can be a spread that has been created by the reader themselves, or it may be a spread that has been developed by someone else. Each position within the spread will be defined, as well as the format of the spread itself. Certain spreads will relate better to certain questions. The smaller the spread (the fewer cards that are used), the easier it will be for a beginning reader to interpret.

A one card spread can be used for any question, as can the traditional ten card Celtic Cross spread. (The Celtic Cross spread is also good to use when the question is more general in nature.) A three card spread can be defined in many ways, and can bring out a great deal of information. The format can be linear, or set in a triangle. Some of the ways that it can be read are: Past/Present/Future, Morning/Noon/Night, Opportunity/Challenge/Outcome, and Issue/Challenge/Action. However you want to define this reading, it is great fun, and will bring out a great deal of information.

A simple four card format that looks at the question/issue from the perspective of the four levels of life is the Elemental Spread. I define the positions here as: East/Spiritual, South/Emotional, West/Physical, and North/Mental. A fifth card can be drawn to represent the Seeker, and placed in the middle of the other four cards (which form a diamond pattern).

Tarot spreads can be found in most Tarot books, as well as on the Internet. There are books specifically devoted to Tarot spreads, such as the Complete Book of Tarot Spreads by Evelin Burger and Johannes Fiebig (Sterling Publishing Company, 1995,1997); and, for those who wish to understand how to create their own Tarot spreads, books such as Designing Your Own Tarot Spreads, by Teresa Michelson.

You have focused in on a specific question or issue, the cards have been shuffled, and the manner of reading (using, or not using, a formal spread) decided upon. Now you need to decide, as a reader, whether to lay the cards face up or face down. This is an individual decision - do whatever you are most comfortable with. I have always chosen to read with the cards face up, because I want to see the larger picture before I begin my reading. Other readers prefer to allow the story to unfold as the cards are turned over. It is up to you to determine what works best for you.

Take a deep breath, exhale, and allow the images on the cards to come to you. Now is your time to shine, as you interpret the cards individually, and as a group. The first thing that you want to do is to take a look at the overall pattern of the spread - which symbols are you drawn to, what do the colors tell you, what kind of flow do the cards have? Is there a predominance of Major Arcana cards? If so, the outcome is largely out of the Seeker's hands, and the reading itself is highly spiritual in nature. What is the balance between the suits? If there is a predominance of one suit, the energy of that suit is predominant in the reading. (In general, the energy of Wands is active, creative, and having to do with personal will power; the energy of Cups is that of the emotional world, the subconscious self, and intuition; the energy of Swords is the energy of intellect and communications; the energy of Pentacles is the energy of finances, work, and the environment around you.) I take this one step farther, in that if a particular suit does not come up in a reading (especially in larger readings), then I feel that the "way out" of the Seeker's dilemma is to be found in that suit. Wherever Aces appear, you are looking at "potential" - at unmanifested energy.

Wherever Court Cards appear, there will be people involved in the issue. If you read with reversals, look at which positions they fall in. Are they in the past? Are they in the present? Are they in the future? If you do not read with reversals (which I do not), work on another method of determining the strength or weakness of a card. Using Elemental Dignities is an excellent choice here.

Where do you begin a reading? At the beginning, of course! Start with the first card. Look at the landscape, the colors, the images, and the symbols. What stands out for you? How does what you see relate to the question the Seeker is asking? If you are reading for someone else, ask them how they feel about the card. I normally tape readings that I do for others, so that they can take the tape home with them. Readings are ripe with emotion - no one is going to remember everything that was said, no matter how important is was. Having a tape of the reading will help your client work through the information that they were presented with. If you are reading for yourself, you may want to either do a tape for yourself, or make notes as you go along. Some readers will choose to wait until the end of the reading to make notes, if they are reading for themselves.

The story begins with the very first card, and winds through the labyrinth of cards to the last card. If a card seems unclear, draw one card from the deck to act as a clarifier, then move on to the next card. If the end card is a Trump (Major Arcana card), there is little the Seeker can do to change the path of the issue. In this case, they need to work on understanding it. If the end card is a Court Card, then other people are involved with the resolution of the issue. If the end card is a Pip (numbered card), then the Seeker can take actions that will change their path.

Above all, a reading is a snapshot of the Seeker's life at a specific place in time. It is a reflection of the energies in their life, and it shows where their opportunities and challenges are. This is their story, a story that will unfold as it should from card to card, each card gaining meaning from the others. Each card holds a basic (traditional) meaning, but each card also holds a meaning that it gains from the cards around it.
When you first begin to read the cards, go through a reading intuitively, speaking what comes through to you from the images in the cards. Then, if you wish, go back and check the "traditional" meaning of the cards. Know that as you do more and more readings, you will develop your own sense of what a card means, and where it is taking you. Keeping a journal of your readings will allow you to see your progress on a very real level, as well as allowing you to see how specific issues develop in your life.

There are many helpful resources for doing readings. Two that I would suggest are the excellent book Tarot For Yourself, by Mary K. Greer, and the Internet site by Tarot author Joan Bunning. The Comparative Tarot e-group on Yahoo Groups provides a wonderful atmosphere for asking questions, as does the forum at Aeclectic Tarot.

Happy reading - and remember to have fun!

How to Read Tea Leaves

Follow this simple 6 step procedure to read tea leaves for yourself or a friend. Tea leaf reading is easy, fun and possibly a little bit enlightening!

Step 1: Make a cup of tea.

Choose a white or light colored teacup. Almost any leaf tea will do nicely. My personal preference is Earl Grey. If avoiding caffeine, you might even choose an herbal variety. The herbal options are delicious: jasmine, peppermint, chamomile... the list goes on and on.
If you do not mind the tiny floating bits, you can open a tea bag and sprinkle the tea into a cup of hot water. A Middle Eastern option is to sprinkle coffee grounds into a cup of coffee.

Step 2: Steep your tea and quiet your mind.

Steeping time is a personal preference. Green and black teas are usually ready in a minute or two, while herbal teas may take longer.

This is a time to quiet your mind and relax. What you are about to exercise is your mental creativity. Pattern recognition and symbol recollection will require focus and concentration. Distracting conversation, music or activity will detract from your experience. As in beginning meditation, attempt to empty your mind of all thoughts.

Step 3: Sip tea while you find your focus.

Once your tea is cool enough, begin sipping. Leaves may be floating, so do the best you can to avoid consuming too many. If you are right-handed, lift your cup with your left. If left-handed, drink with your right. If ambidextrous, reach for your cup, stop, and then use the other hand.

Now that you are quiet and relaxed, identify the issue foremost in your mind. In meditation practice, one attempts to empty the mind -- blocking out all thoughts. As you attempt to think of nothing in particular, is there a stubborn thought that keeps returning to your attention? If so, that is the subject of this reading. Focus on that thought.

If nothing in particular comes to mind, then this will be a general tea leaf reading. Focus on your breath and the taste of the tea.

Leave a small amount of tea at the bottom of your cup

.

Step 4: Swirl three times and dump.

Hold your nearly empty teacup in your hand and give it three good swirls. The tea leaves will disperse around the interior of cup. Gently dump out the remaining liquid by turning your teacup over into a saucer.

Wait at least three breaths before turning your cup back over. You are ready to begin reading your tea leaves!

Step 5: Identify symbols and jot them down.

Tea leaf reading is a highly personal and subjective process. Because abstract pattern recognition keys into our subconscious, self-analysis produces the most relevant reading. One person may see an egg, while another sees a beetle in the same spot. Tea leaf reading is very much like a Rorschach (Ink Blot) Test. We are most likely to recognize symbols having a bearing on or connection with the matter at hand. Therefore, you are the most qualified person to read your own tea leaves.

If your cup has a handle, begin there and read clockwise. If your cup has no handle, begin reading from 12 o'clock. Make a notation of the first symbol you see. Mentally divide the cup into three sections: rim, middle and base. The rim area is above the tea level when you first poured your tea. The base is the level of tea left before you dumped out the remainder. The middle section is the area between the rim and bottom. Note where the symbol is located and if it is next to another symbol. Note whether you see bubbles, twigs or droplets in your cup. Work with quiet concentration and take your time.

Step 6: Create your tea leaf reading.

Translating symbols into meaning is just as personal and subjective as their identification. Individual language, cultural exposure, experience, knowledge and mental state contribute to interpretation of symbols. For example, the letter "K" might first bring to mind your friend Kurt rather than your sister Kirstin. Next to each symbol you wrote down, jot down the meaning that comes to mind first.

Again, abstract pattern recognition keys into our subconscious, so self-analysis produces the most relevant reading. You are the most qualified person to read your own tea leaves. That being said, this site provides an extensive symbol lexicon to assist you in identifying and recalling symbols.

The first symbol you saw represents your dominant character or someone near or influential. Symbols in the rim section apply to this moment in time. The middle section represents the near future -- usually no longer than a fortnight. Both the rim and middle section represent influences in your outcome. The base of your cup represents the ultimate answer or conclusion.

Summary

So I hope you enjoyed this lesson on Avoiding Accidents. I really wanted to use my experience with Premonitions to help you learn that these abilities can be used by anyone.

It's like doing exercise which builds muscles. The more you practice premonitional techniques, the more they will work for you.

And don't forget that we are really talking about changing the probabilities of the future events happening. You can change these events, even though it might take a lot of force of will.

Some events like the 911 tragedy are so huge that you will probably not be able to impact them, but personal life events can definitely be altered depending upon how much you want to do so.

Use these techniques and Stay Safe!